Simplified Solution Approach

To SLEEP

DISORDERS

The Ultimate Sleep Solution: Break Free from Insomnia and Fatigue, and Embrace a Healthier, More Vibrant You

Dr QUENTIN GLYN

Table Of Contents

CHAPTER ONE

Sleep Disorders

For many people in today's hectic environment, getting enough sleep has become a luxury. Millions of people worldwide are affected by sleep problems, which are becoming more common as our lives get busier and more entwined with technology.

In order to assist readers in better understanding and managing sleep issues and to promote general health and well-being, this book attempts to provide a straightforward solution approach.

Recognizing The Value Of Sleep:

A vital component of life, sleep is essential for maintaining one's physical, mental, and emotional health. The body performs vital functions like hormone management, memory consolidation, and tissue repair when we sleep. Stronger immune systems, better cognitive performance, and emotional resilience are all associated with getting enough sleep.

The Effects Of Sleep On Physical And Mental Health:

Inadequate sleep has far-reaching consequences. Chronic sleep deprivation has been linked to a higher risk of heart disease, obesity, diabetes, and mental health disorders, among other health problems. Inadequate sleep may also negatively impact memory, decision-making abilities, and cognitive function, which can lower productivity and lower quality of life.

Typical Myths Regarding Sleep:

Dispelling myths about sleep is essential to gaining a thorough understanding of its significance. Many individuals undervalue the importance of regular sleep patterns because they think that sporadic disruptions to sleep are insignificant. This book will dispel popular misconceptions and highlight the cumulative effects of insufficient sleep on long-term health.

An Overview Of Sleep Issues:

Sleep disorders are a wide spectrum of problems that interfere with the body's normal circadian rhythm. These conditions may be divided into four groups: circadian rhythm disorders, parasomnias, insomnia, and sleep apnea. It is essential to comprehend the unique features of every condition in order to make an accurate diagnosis and provide successful therapy.

Categories And Types:

There will be a thorough examination of the many kinds of sleep problems, their signs, and their underlying causes. Readers will learn more about common diseases such as restless legs syndrome, obstructive sleep apnea, and primary insomnia. Having a clear categorization system would help in addressing certain sleep-related issues with remedies.

Frequency And Social Effects:

Sleep issues are becoming more common and impacting people of all ages and backgrounds. The effects on society are significant; they lead to higher healthcare expenses, worse productivity at work, and an increase in accidents because of cognitive impairment. The need for practical remedies is emphasized by being aware of the wider effects of sleep disturbances.

The Requirement Of A Simplified Approach To Solutions:

The conventional approaches to treating sleep disturbances may be intimidating and complicated. This book promotes a solution-focused approach, offering doable tactics that readers may simply apply to their daily lives. The goal is to provide clear answers and demystify sleep science so that people may take charge of their sleep health.

Problems With Current Treatment Approaches:

Many of the problems with the current treatment approaches are related to cost, side effects, and accessibility. The book will discuss these drawbacks and provide substitute strategies that put an emphasis on sustainability, affordability, and simplicity.

The Book's Objective:

The goal of "Restful Nights" is to provide readers with a thorough understanding of sleep problems and how to avoid and treat them. The goal of the book is to close the gap between scientific understanding and doable, practical methods for getting a good night's sleep that revitalizes the body by offering a simple solution approach.

The book will explore certain sleep disorders, lifestyle variables that affect sleep, and evidence-based methods for improving sleep hygiene in later chapters.

CHAPTER TWO

Basics Of Sleep

The basics of sleep: Essentially a complicated physiological process, sleep is vital to general health and wellness. It is distinguished by a lowered level of awareness and attentiveness, along with certain alterations in brain activity and physiological processes. Sleep is essential for several critical processes, such as emotional control, memory consolidation, and physical repair.

Phases And Cycles Of Sleep:

Sleep Stages: Non-rapid Eye Movement (NREM) sleep and Rapid Eye Movement (REM) sleep are the two primary categories into which sleep is usually classified.

NREM Sleep: This kind of sleep, which is broken down into three phases (N1, N2, and N3), is linked to the first phase of the transition from waking to deep sleep. N1 is the lightest stage of sleep, N2 is a little bit deeper, and N3, the deepest stage of sleep, is the most important for physical recovery.

Vibrant dreaming happens during REM sleep, which is crucial for learning, mood management, and cognitive processes.

Sleep Cycles: A whole sleep cycle lasts around 90 to 110 minutes and includes both REM and NREM sleep. Multiple cycles occur throughout a full night's sleep, and each one supports a distinct facet of both physical and mental recovery.

The Circadian Rhythms:

Definition: Internal biological processes known as circadian rhythms are regulated by light and darkness and follow an approximately 24-hour cycle. The circadian rhythm is essential for controlling the cycle of sleep and wakefulness.

Function in Sleep: The brain's suprachiasmatic nucleus controls the body's internal clock, which synchronizes a number of physiological functions with the outside world. Sleep problems may be exacerbated by circadian rhythm disruptions, such as shift work or inconsistent sleep habits.

Numerous neurotransmitters and hormones are involved in the regulation of sleep, and their functions are crucial.

Melatonin: A hormone that aids in controlling the sleep-wake cycle, melatonin is produced by the pineal gland. Exposure to light affects its production, with levels usually increasing in the evening to promote slumber.

Adenosine: This neurotransmitter encourages tiredness by building up in the brain during waking hours. One typical stimulant that delays the onset of tiredness is caffeine. It does this by inhibiting adenosine receptors.

Gamma-aminobutyric acid (GABA) and serotonin are two neurotransmitters that support the preservation of NREM sleep and control the structure of sleep.

The Brain's Function In Regulating Sleep:

Brain regions Involved: The regulation of sleep is significantly influenced by a number of brain regions, including the brainstem, thalamus, and hypothalamus.

The hypothalamus regulates the release of hormones such as melatonin and serves as the body's internal clock.

The thalamus controls the flow of sensory data, which lowers sensitivity to outside stimuli while you're sleeping.

Brainstem: Regulates respiration and heart rate, among other fundamental physiological processes, while you sleep.

An understanding of the complex interactions between these elements serves as a basis for treating sleep problems. A comprehensive strategy includes dietary adjustments, good sleep hygiene habits, and sometimes, medicinal treatments. People may strive toward getting restorative and rejuvenating sleep by identifying and treating disturbances in circadian rhythms, neurochemical balance, and sleep architecture.

CHAPTER THREE
Recognizing Sleep Issues

Maintaining general health and well-being depends on diagnosing and treating sleep disturbances. Sleep disturbances may significantly affect one's physical and mental health as well as emotional and mental well-being, among other facets of life.

This talk will cover the idea of diagnosing sleep disorders, identify common sleep disorders such as narcolepsy, sleep apnea, insomnia, and restless legs syndrome, and go into the diagnostic methods and instruments used in this area.

Recognizing Sleep Issues:

Clinical Assessment:

Finding sleep problems usually starts with a thorough clinical assessment. This entails speaking with a healthcare provider about the patient's lifestyle, sleep habits, and medical background.

Self-Reporting by Patients:

Patients who are encouraged to maintain a sleep journal may learn a great deal about their sleeping patterns, habits, and any recurrent problems. Information about wake-up and bedtime schedules, sleep quality, and other sleep-influencing variables could be included in this.

Identifying Typical Sleep Disorders:

Sleeplessness:

Difficulties getting to sleep, remaining asleep, or having non-restorative sleep are all signs of insomnia. Numerous things, including stress, worry, and certain medical disorders, might contribute to it.

Apnea during sleep:

Breathing irregularities while you sleep are a defining feature of sleep apnea. Obstructive sleep apnea (OSA) and central sleep apnea (CSA) are the two primary forms. The more prevalent kind of OSA is brought on by excessive throat muscular relaxation.

Narcolepsy

A neurological condition called narcolepsy interferes with the brain's capacity to control sleep-wake cycles. People who have narcolepsy may go into abrupt, unpredictable sleep phases throughout the day.

RLS, or restless legs syndrome:

RLS is characterized by painful leg sensations that are often accompanied by a strong desire to move the legs. These sensations might interfere with sleep and usually become worse when you're not moving.

Instruments And Methods For Diagnosis:

Research on Sleep:

A thorough sleep study called polysomnography (PSG) keeps track of several physiological variables while a person is asleep. It comprises assessments of heart rate, respiratory function, muscular activity, eye movement, and brain activity.

Testing for sleep apnea at home (HSAT):

Portable equipment may be used in a home environment to monitor heart rate, oxygen levels, and breathing patterns during sleep in order to diagnose sleep apnea. For certain patients, this method is more convenient.

Assessments And Questionnaires:

Epworth Scale of Sleepiness:

People are asked to judge how likely they are to fall asleep in different scenarios in order to measure daytime drowsiness. It aids in determining how drowsy a person is.

The PSQI (Pittsburgh Sleep Quality Index):

The PSQI is a self-report tool used to evaluate sleep disruptions and quality over a period of one month. It addresses a number of topics related to sleep, such as length, latency, and disruptions.

International Study Group Rating Scale for Restless Legs Syndrome:

Restless legs syndrome is diagnosed and its severity is evaluated using this scale. It assesses how often and how severe RLS symptoms are.

A comprehensive strategy that incorporates clinical assessment, patient self-reporting, and the use of specialist diagnostic instruments is necessary to identify sleep disorders. Developing successful treatment regimens for common sleep disorders such as narcolepsy, insomnia, sleep apnea, and restless legs syndrome requires an understanding of these conditions. Accurate diagnosis and treatment of sleep disorders depend heavily on diagnostic instruments, such as questionnaires and sleep tests.

CHAPTER FOUR

Factors In Lifestyle That Impact Sleep

Of course! Let's explore the several lifestyle elements that may have a big influence on how well you sleep, such as nutrition, exercise, good sleep hygiene, and setting up a sleep-friendly atmosphere.

Dietary Influence On Sleep:

1. Foods that Aid with Sleep:

Foods High in Tryptophan: The amino acid tryptophan is a precursor to the sleep-regulating chemicals melatonin and serotonin. Tryptophan is found in foods including turkey, dairy, almonds, and seeds, and it may help you sleep better.

Complex Carbohydrates: Meals that raise serotonin levels, such as whole grains and legumes, might help you feel more at peace before bed.

Foods High in Magnesium: Magnesium promotes calmness by relaxing muscles and nerves. Nuts, whole grains, and leafy greens are excellent sources.

2. Meals that Prevent Sleep:

Caffeine: A stimulant that may interfere with sleep, caffeine is found in coffee, tea, chocolate, and certain drugs. Restrict your consumption, particularly in the afternoon and evening.

High-fat and spicy foods: These might upset your stomach and interfere with your ability to fall asleep. It's best to steer clear of large meals just before bed.

The Function Of Exercise:

1. Exercise and the Quality of Sleep:

Exercise Timing: Although regular exercise helps improve sleep, it may also be stimulating just before bed. Early in the day, try to get in some moderate activity.

Over time, establishing a regular exercise regimen might help normalize sleep patterns.

Hygiene Practices For Sleep:

1.   Creating   a   Sleep-Conducive Environment:

Purchasing a comfy mattress and pillows helps to maintain optimal spinal alignment and lessens pain.

Ideal Room Temperature and Darkness: Sleeping is best in a room that is cold and dark. Think about keeping the temperature moderate and using blackout curtains.

Minimize Light and Noise: To establish a peaceful sleeping environment, minimize distracting components like light and noise.

2. Creating Regular Sleep Schedules:

Maintain a Regular Sleep Schedule: The body's internal clock is regulated when you go to bed and get up at the same time each day.

Limiting Naps: Taking frequent, extended naps might disrupt your sleep at night, while short naps can be helpful.

Establish a calming ritual before going to bed to let your body know when it's time to unwind. Activities like reading or having a warm bath might fall under this category.

Improving lifestyle variables may make a big difference in the quality of sleep. People may improve their overall quality of sleep by adopting appropriate sleep hygiene habits, making thoughtful dietary choices, getting regular exercise, and setting up a sleep-friendly atmosphere. It's critical to understand how these variables are related to one another and how living a holistic lifestyle may improve sleep and general well-being.

It is essential to seek additional examination and help from a healthcare expert if sleep disorders continue.

CHAPTER FIVE

Behavioral And Cognitive Methods

Sleep disorders are widespread problems that may have a major negative influence on a person's general well-being. They include a variety of ailments that impair both the amount and quality of sleep.

Cognitive and behavioral therapies (CBT) have become the most well-researched and successful therapy option for treating sleep disturbances among other treatments. The concept of Cognitive and Behavioral Approaches will be covered in great detail in this article, with a particular emphasis on

Cognitive Behavioral Therapy for Insomnia (CBT-I), addressing negative thought patterns, creating healthy sleep habits, practicing relaxation, and using cognitive strategies to manage sleep disorders.

1. Cognitive Behavioral Therapy For Insomnia (CBT-I): Cognitive behavioral therapy for insomnia (CBT-I) is a goal-oriented, organized therapeutic technique created especially for those who experience sleeplessness. Through the modification of maladaptive thinking patterns and behaviors that lead to sleep problems, CBT-I seeks to address the underlying causes of insomnia, in contrast to medication-based therapies. Usually involving many sessions with a qualified

therapist, the treatment combines a number of behavioral and cognitive strategies.

2. Resolving Negative Thinking Patterns: Also known as cognitive distortions, negative thinking patterns have a major role in the emergence and maintenance of sleep problems. The goal of CBT-I is to recognize and confront these false beliefs about sleep. Strategies like cognitive restructuring assist people in reframing unfavorable ideas into more realistic and balanced viewpoints, fostering a more positive outlook that improves sleep quality.

3. Creating And Sustaining Healthy Sleep Behaviors: A key element of CBT-I is the development and upkeep of healthy sleep behaviors or sleep hygiene. This entails teaching people the value of adhering to regular sleep patterns, setting up a sleeping-friendly atmosphere, and avoiding behaviors that can interfere with sleep, such as consuming too much coffee or spending time on screens just before bed. CBT-I attempts to increase the length and quality of sleep overall by establishing these behaviors.

4. Relaxation Strategies: To lessen the physiological and psychological arousal that might prevent sleep, CBT-I includes relaxation strategies. Common relaxation techniques used in CBT-I include progressive muscle relaxation, guided imagery, and deep breathing exercises. By assisting people in reaching a state of mental and physical tranquility, these strategies facilitate the smoother transition from awake to sound sleep.

5. Meditation, Yoga, And Mindfulness: Mind-body techniques are integral to CBT-I. These include meditation, yoga, and mindfulness. Engaging in these activities may help you de-stress, become more self-aware, and relax. By incorporating mindfulness into everyday activities, people might better handle stresses that would otherwise lead to sleep problems by being more aware of their thoughts and emotions.

6. Cognitive Methods For Treating Sleep Problems: CBT-I uses a variety of cognitive techniques to target different components of sleep problems. These might include using sensory control strategies to reinforce the relationship between the bedroom and sleep, as well as cognitive restructuring, which entails questioning and altering unfavorable ideas about sleep. Through focusing on cognitive components, CBT-I enables people to actively manage their sleep issues.

In conclusion, behavioral and cognitive approaches, especially cognitive behavioral therapy for insomnia, provide a thorough and easy-to-understand way to treat sleep problems. Through the use of relaxation methods, integration of cognitive strategies, targeting negative thinking patterns, and promotion of good sleep habits, CBT-I offers people useful tools to enhance their general well-being and reclaim control over their sleep. Accepting these methods gives people the ability to create long-lasting adjustments that lead to more satisfying and peaceful sleep.

CHAPTER SIX

Technological Remedies

A large percentage of people worldwide suffer from sleep disturbances, which have an adverse effect on their physical and mental health. Thankfully, technological developments have opened the door for creative approaches to problems with sleep. This article examines a technologically-enhanced, streamlined method of treating sleep problems.

Wearable Technology To Monitor Sleep:

Fitness trackers and smartwatches are examples of wearable technology that have become essential for tracking sleep habits.

These gadgets measure movement, heart rate, and even ambient elements using sensors to provide insightful data on the quality of sleep. In order to enhance general sleep health, users may better understand their sleep cycles, spot disruptions, and make educated modifications.

Tracking Trends And Patterns In Sleep:

In addition, advanced monitoring systems that track trends and patterns in sleep are examples of technological solutions. These systems often interpret data from several sources, including wearable technology and specialized sleep sensors, using artificial intelligence (AI) algorithms. Through the process of recognizing recurring trends and deviations, people may discover possible problems related to their sleep and work with medical specialists to develop focused solutions.

Apps & Programs For Sleep:

The use of smartphone apps made especially for managing sleep has increased. Features like guided interventions, individualized sleep suggestions, and sleep monitoring are included in these applications. Certain applications use the concepts of cognitive-behavioral therapy for insomnia (CBT-I), offering users research-backed methods for enhancing sleep hygiene and encouraging improved sleep patterns.

Sleep Aids And Guided Meditations:

A plethora of applications and digital spaces provide guided meditations and relaxation methods to assist people in decompressing before going to bed. These tools often use soothing stories, aural cues, and visual assistance to create a relaxed atmosphere that promotes sleep. Applications that produce white noise and natural noises may also provide a calming atmosphere, blocking out outside noise and encouraging a calmer sleeping environment.

New Developments In Sleep Medicine Technologies:

With the advent of cutting-edge technology, the area of sleep medicine is still developing. Among the significant advancements are:

a. Neurofeedback: This technique trains people to attain more ideal sleep patterns by using electroencephalogram (EEG) technology to deliver real-time feedback on brainwave activity.

b. VR Therapy: Applications for VR are being investigated as potential therapeutic tools to treat sleep issues. It is possible to create virtual spaces that promote calmness and reduce tension, which will enhance the quality of your sleep.

c. Smart Bedding and Mattresses: Continuous monitoring of sleep quality is made possible by the integration of sensors into bedding and mattresses. These gadgets can monitor motion, change the hardness of the mattress, and even provide customized sleep reports.

The use of technology solutions in the treatment of sleep problems provides a thorough yet streamlined method. People may now actively participate in understanding and enhancing their sleep health thanks to wearable technology, monitoring systems, guided meditations, sleep applications, and new developments in sleep medicine. There is yet hope for new creative and practical approaches to treating sleep-related problems as long as technology keeps developing.

CHAPTER SEVEN

Nutritional Measures

Dietary Techniques To Improve Sleep:

1. A well-rounded diet

• Eating a healthy, well-balanced diet full of vital elements, such as vitamins and minerals, may improve sleep quality and enhance general health. Lean meats, whole grains, fruits, vegetables, and healthy fats are all part of a diet that offers the nutrition needed for all of the body's processes, including sleep.

2. Setting Mealtime Routines:

• Setting regular mealtimes supports a regular sleep-wake cycle by regulating the body's internal clock. Large meals should be avoided just before bed to avoid pain and indigestion, which may interfere with sleep.

Foods That Encourage The Production Of Melatonin:

1. Rich in Tryptophan Foods:

• The amino acid tryptophan is a precursor to the neurotransmitters melatonin and serotonin, which control mood and sleep. Tryptophan-rich foods include dairy products, nuts, seeds, turkey, and chicken.

2. Rich in Melatonin Foods:

• The hormone that controls sleep-wake cycles, melatonin, is found naturally in several meals. Pomegranates, tomatoes, grapes, and cherries are a few examples. Including these in your diet might help to encourage the generation of melatonin naturally.

Supplemental Nutrition To Promote Sleep:

1. Supplements with melatonin:

• Supplemental melatonin is often used to treat sleep disturbances. However, because taking too much melatonin might have negative consequences, it's important to use them sparingly and under a doctor's supervision.

2. The mineral magnesium

• Magnesium helps relax muscles, which may improve sleep quality. For people who are deficient, foods high in magnesium, such as leafy green vegetables, nuts, and seeds, as well as magnesium supplements, may be helpful.

3. B complex vitamin:

• B vitamins are involved in the formation of melatonin, including B6, B9 (folate), and B12. Foods high in B vitamins, such as fish, chicken, leafy greens, and fortified cereals, may help ensure an adequate intake.

The Brain-Gut Relationship:

1. Microbiota and Sleep:

• A considerable correlation between sleep and gut flora has been shown by emerging studies. The gut microbiota's diversity and balance may have a beneficial effect on sleep patterns. Gut health may be supported by consuming prebiotics, which are present in foods like garlic, onions, and bananas, and probiotics, which are present in yogurt, kefir, and fermented foods.

2. Digestive Health's Effect on Sleep:

• Digestion problems may cause sleep disturbances, including GERD and irritable bowel syndrome (IBS). Better sleep may result from avoiding trigger foods, maintaining a balanced gut microbiota, and controlling digestive issues with dietary changes.

A comprehensive strategy for treating sleep problems must take nutritional therapies into account as a critical component. Although there isn't a single, effective treatment, a balanced diet, an emphasis on foods that promote sleep, and gut health support may all help with better quality sleep. A trained dietitian or other healthcare expert should always be consulted in order to customize dietary treatments to each person's requirements and address any underlying health issues.

CHAPTER EIGHT

Alternative And Herbal Medicines

Compared to traditional pharmaceuticals, herbal and alternative medicines are becoming more and more well-liked as a comprehensive and often softer way of treating sleep problems.

While it's important to speak with medical specialists before beginning any new therapy, a number of complementary and alternative treatments, including herbal medicines, have shown promise in improving sleep quality. Here is a thorough summary of some important ideas in this field:

Herbal Treatments For Insomnia

Valerian:

Overview: One of the most well-known natural sleep aids is valerian root. It is thought to interact with brain chemicals that control relaxation and sleep.

Efficacy: Based on some research, valerian may shorten the time it takes to fall asleep and enhance the quality of sleep. Results might differ, however, and additional study is required.

Chamomile:

Overview: Chamomile is well-known for its relaxing qualities and is often drunk as tea.

Antioxidants and substances with a slight sedative effect are present in it.

Efficacy: Although chamomile has long been used to induce calmness and sleep, there isn't much scientific proof to back up this claim. If you have mild sleep disturbances, it might work better.

Lavender:

Overview: Lavender is thought to have calming effects on the nervous system when consumed in various forms, such as tea or essential oil.

Efficacy: According to certain research, smelling lavender or applying lavender essential oil can enhance relaxation, lower anxiety, and improve the quality of sleep.

a passionflower

Overview: The plant passionflower has long been used to treat sleeplessness and anxiety.

Efficacy: Studies suggest that passionflower may help enhance the quality of sleep and have a mild sedative effect, but more research is required to confirm this.

Traditional Chinese Medicine And Acupuncture:

Acupuncture

Overview: One of the main tenets of Traditional Chinese Medicine (TCM) is acupuncture, which involves balancing the body's energy flow (Qi) by putting tiny needles into particular points.

Efficacy: By encouraging relaxation and balancing the body's energy, some research indicates that acupuncture may help enhance the quality of sleep and lessen the symptoms of insomnia.

Chinese Herbal Medicine:

Overview: Traditional Chinese medicine (TCM) uses a variety of herbal formulas to treat bodily imbalances, including sleep-related ones.

Effectiveness: Traditional medicine has utilized certain herbal mixtures, like Suan Zao Ren Tang, to treat insomnia. The effectiveness of these herbal formulations is still being studied scientifically.

The Effectiveness Of Other Alternative Therapies:

Meditation with mindfulness:

Overview: The goal of mindfulness exercises, such as meditation, is to increase awareness of the present moment, which may lessen stress and encourage relaxation.

Efficacy: Research indicates that by addressing stress and encouraging relaxation, mindfulness meditation may enhance the quality of sleep and lessen the symptoms of insomnia.

Yoga:

Overview: Yoga enhances general well-being by combining physical postures, breath control, and meditation.

Effectiveness: A few yoga poses, particularly those that emphasize breathing and relaxation, may be able to reduce the symptoms of insomnia and enhance the quality of your sleep.

Insomnia Treatment with Cognitive Behavioral Therapy (CBT-I):

Overview: CBT-I is an organized therapeutic method that focuses on the attitudes, actions, and routines that lead to sleeplessness.

Efficacy: Research has demonstrated that CBT-I, which targets underlying behavioral and psychological issues, is a very successful treatment for insomnia.

In summary, those looking for a comprehensive approach to treating sleep disorders have a wide range of options with herbal remedies and alternative therapies. Even though some of these interventions have yielded encouraging results, it is important to approach them with the knowledge that each person will respond differently. Seeking advice from medical specialists and integrating these treatments into a thorough sleep management strategy could yield a more individualized and successful outcome.

CHAPTER NINE
Developing A Customized Sleep Schedule

In order to address sleep disorders, developing a personalized sleep plan is essential because it enables a focused and customized approach to enhancing the quality of sleep.

This plan calls for combining several strategies, customizing responses to meet the needs of each individual, setting and monitoring sleep objectives, and putting long-term maintenance plans into action.

1. Evaluation Of Personal Needs:

• Sleep Assessment: Start by performing a comprehensive evaluation of the person's sleeping habits, patterns, and ambient factors. This could entail using wearable technology, keeping a sleep journal, or, if needed, getting sleep studies done.

• Determining the Root Causes: Determine which particular elements—such as stress, lifestyle decisions, health issues, or environmental factors—are causing sleep disturbances.

2. Combining Various Methods:

• Cognitive-behavioral therapy for Insomnia (CBT-I): Use evidence-based treatments that target the maladaptive thought and behavior patterns linked to insomnia, such as CBT-I.

• Sleep Hygiene: Adopt appropriate sleep hygiene measures, such as sticking to a regular sleep schedule, setting up a cozy sleeping space, and refraining from stimulants right before bed.

• Relaxation Techniques: To lessen stress and anxiety, incorporate relaxation techniques like progressive muscle relaxation, deep breathing, or mindfulness meditation.

3. Customizing Solutions To Meet Every Need:

• Customizing Sleep Environment: Make changes to the sleeping environment to meet personal preferences. Some examples include minimizing light and noise, selecting the ideal mattress and pillows, and adjusting the temperature of the room.

• Including Physical Activity: Create an exercise regimen that enhances general well-being and may have a favorable effect on sleep. To prevent interfering with sleep, exercise schedules and intensities should be customized.

4. Setting And Monitoring Sleep Objectives:

• Creating Achievable Short- and Long-Term Sleep Goals: Work together to create realistic sleep objectives. Objectives could be hitting a daily sleep threshold, cutting down on the amount of time it takes to fall asleep, or enhancing the quality of sleep.

• Tracking Progress: To keep an eye on things, use sleep-tracking apps and make frequent check-ins. In light of feedback and modifications to sleep patterns, modify the sleep plan as necessary.

5. Strategies For Long-Term Maintenance:

• Lifestyle Modifications: Promote long-term adjustments to one's routine that promote sound sleep, such as stress management, sticking to a regular sleep schedule, and minimizing screen time before bed.

• Frequent Follow-Ups: Arrange for regular follow-up appointments to evaluate continuing sleep patterns and promptly address any new issues that may arise.

• Adaptability: Be aware that as your needs for sleep change over time, your sleep schedule should be flexible enough to adjust for stressors, life changes, or changes in your health.

A thorough and efficient framework for treating sleep disorders is provided by a customized sleep plan that combines various techniques, adjusts solutions to meet the needs of the individual, sets and monitors sleep goals, and includes long-term maintenance techniques. This all-encompassing strategy not only addresses pressing issues but also promotes long-term gains in overall well-being and the quality of sleep.

Conclusion

In summary, treating and managing sleep disorders calls for a customized, multifaceted strategy. By understanding the key concepts discussed in this simplified solution approach, individuals can empower themselves to take control of their sleep and make positive changes to improve their overall well-being.

Recap Of Key Concepts:

Understanding Sleep Disorders: It's crucial to recognize the diverse nature of sleep disorders, which can range from insomnia and sleep apnea to restless leg syndrome and narcolepsy. Each disorder has its unique characteristics and underlying causes, making it essential to identify specific symptoms for accurate diagnosis.

Lifestyle Modifications: Adopting healthy sleep habits is a fundamental aspect of managing sleep disorders. This includes maintaining a consistent sleep schedule, creating a comfortable sleep environment, and incorporating relaxation techniques before bedtime. Lifestyle modifications may also involve dietary adjustments and regular exercise to promote overall health.

Cognitive Behavioral Therapy for Insomnia (CBT-I): CBT-I is a proven therapeutic approach for addressing insomnia. By addressing negative thought patterns and behaviors related to sleep, individuals can restructure their attitudes toward sleep and develop healthier sleep patterns. This evidence-based therapy is often recommended as a first-line treatment for chronic insomnia.

Medical Interventions: In some cases, medical interventions may be necessary. This can range from prescription medications to devices like continuous positive airway pressure (CPAP) machines for sleep apnea. It's crucial for individuals to work closely with healthcare professionals to determine the most appropriate and effective medical interventions for their specific sleep disorder.

Monitoring and Evaluation: Regularly monitoring sleep patterns and evaluating the effectiveness of implemented strategies are essential for long-term success. Keeping a sleep diary, using wearable devices, or undergoing sleep studies can provide valuable insights into the progress made and identify areas that may require further attention.

Empowering Readers To Take Control Of Their Sleep:

Empowerment begins with education. By understanding the various aspects of sleep and sleep disorders, readers can make informed decisions about their lifestyle, and habits, and when to seek professional help. It's crucial to recognize that taking control of one's sleep is a gradual process that involves commitment and consistency.

Educate Themselves: Continuously seek information about sleep, its importance, and common sleep disorders. Understanding the impact of sleep on overall health can motivate individuals to prioritize and invest in their sleep hygiene.

Adopt Healthy Sleep Habits: Incorporate the principles of good sleep hygiene into daily routines. This includes maintaining a regular sleep schedule, creating a comfortable sleep environment, and engaging in relaxing activities before bedtime.

Self-Monitoring: Keep track of sleep patterns, noting any changes or patterns that may indicate a sleep disorder. Self-monitoring can provide valuable data to share with healthcare professionals during consultations.

Seek Support: Share experiences and concerns with friends, family, or support groups. Building a support network can provide emotional encouragement and practical advice for managing sleep-related challenges.

Encouragement For Seeking Professional Guidance When Needed:

While self-help strategies are valuable, there are instances where professional guidance is crucial. Encouraging readers to seek help when needed is an integral part of this solution approach.

Recognizing Limitations: Acknowledge that self-help strategies may have limitations, especially in complex cases or when dealing with severe sleep disorders. Professional guidance ensures a comprehensive assessment and tailored interventions.

Consulting Healthcare Professionals: If sleep problems persist or worsen, readers are encouraged to consult healthcare professionals such as primary care physicians, sleep specialists, or mental health professionals. Timely intervention can prevent the exacerbation of sleep disorders and associated health risks.

Diagnostic Assessments: Professional assessments, including sleep studies and diagnostic evaluations, are crucial for accurate diagnosis.

This allows healthcare providers to recommend targeted interventions based on the specific nature of the sleep disorder.

Customized Treatment Plans: Professionals can create personalized treatment plans that may include a combination of cognitive-behavioral therapy, medication, and lifestyle adjustments. This tailored approach increases the likelihood of successful intervention.

In conclusion, addressing sleep disorders is a journey that involves self-empowerment, education, and, when necessary, seeking professional guidance.

By combining these elements, individuals can take proactive steps toward achieving restful and rejuvenating sleep, ultimately enhancing their overall quality of life.

THE END